Easy Breakfast Ideas For Weight Loss For Beginners

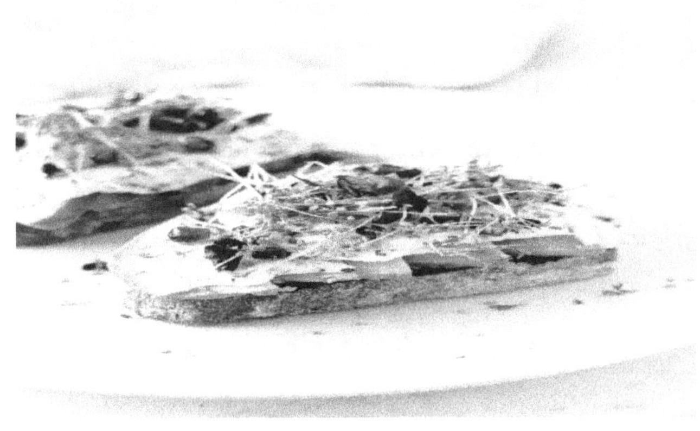

Healthy & Delicious Breakfast Recipes

To Get You Started On Your Weight

Loss Journey

Vanessa Owens

TABLE OF CONTENTS

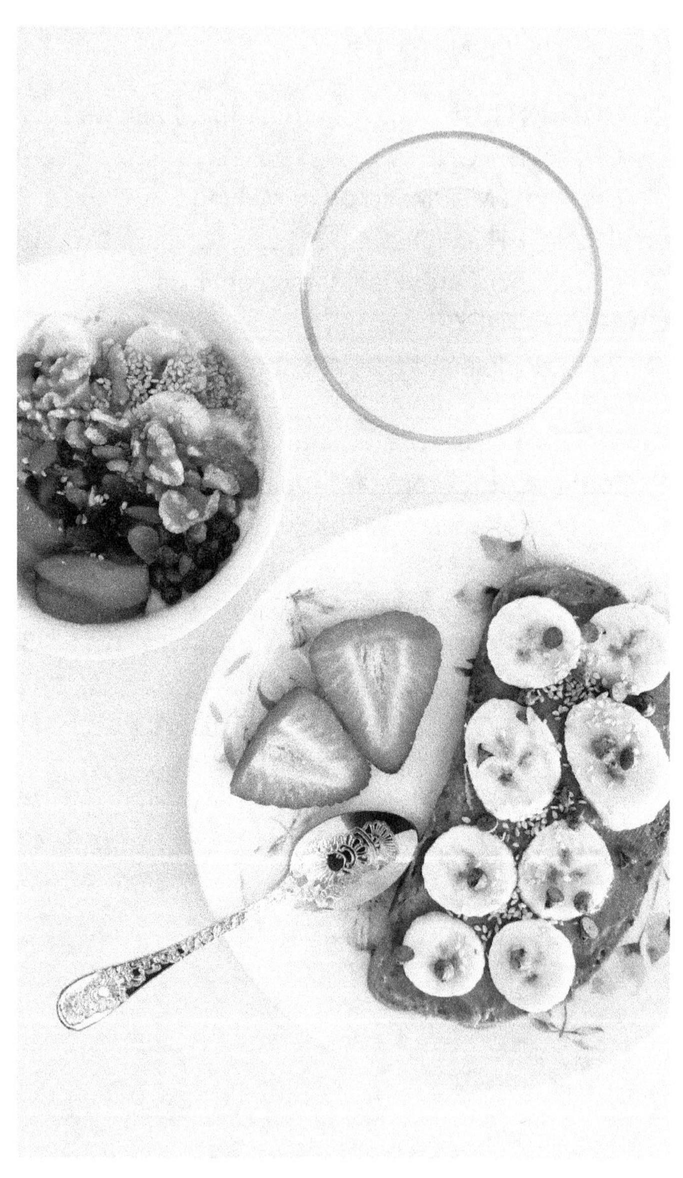

GRATITUDE SPEECH

Ladies and Gentlemen,

I am sincerely grateful for your choice in picking up my book. The support from readers like you means the world to me, and I'm truly honored that you've taken the time to explore the pages I've poured my heart and soul into.

Your decision to read my work is not just a personal victory but a shared journey. Every reader adds a unique perspective, and I'm eager to hear your thoughts. Your feedback is invaluable, and I encourage you to share your honest review. Whether it's a few words or a detailed reflection, your insights help not only me but also potential readers who rely on the experiences of others.

Writing is a labor of love, and your engagement with my book brings it to life. I'm immensely thankful for the opportunity to share this literary adventure with you, and I look forward to hearing about your own journey through the pages.

Thank you for being a part of this incredible voyage, and I hope my words resonate with you as much as your support resonates with me.

Warm regards,

Vanessa Owens.

INTRODUCTION

In the bustling city of Sunriseville, where the aroma of fresh coffee and the sizzle of bacon filled the air, lived Vanessa Owens, a nutrition enthusiast with a passion for creating easy and healthy breakfasts. One day, as she navigated the challenges of maintaining a balanced diet in her own life, inspiration struck her like a ray of morning sunlight.

Motivated to share her discoveries, Vanessa Owens embarked on a culinary journey, experimenting with nutritious ingredients and crafting delicious breakfast recipes tailored for weight loss. The result? A collection of easy breakfast ideas that not only fueled the body but also ignited the taste buds.

In her book, "Easy Breakfast Ideas for Weight Loss for beginners," Vanessa Owens invites readers to join her on a flavorful adventure.

From mouthwatering smoothie bowls bursting with antioxidants to savory egg muffins that redefine on-the-go breakfasts, each recipe is a testament to the belief that healthy eating doesn't have to be bland or complicated.

As readers flip through the pages, they discover not just a cookbook, but a guide to a lifestyle change. Vanessa Owens weaves in tips on portion control, mindful eating, and the science behind the ingredients, making "Easy Breakfast Ideas for Weight Loss for beginners" a holistic approach to weight management.

In a world where time is a scarce commodity, Vanessa's easy breakfast ideas become a beacon of hope for those striving to shed pounds without sacrificing flavor. The book resonates with anyone seeking a practical and sustainable path to a healthier life, reminding them that the journey to weight loss can begin with a simple, satisfying breakfast.

CHAPTER ONE

Breakfast Mistakes You're Making

One common breakfast mistake is skipping it altogether. Many people underestimate the importance of breakfast and either rush through their mornings without eating or intentionally skip the meal, thinking it will help with weight loss.

Skipping breakfast deprives the body of essential nutrients and sets the stage for overeating later in the day. It can lead to decreased energy levels, poor concentration, and increased cravings for unhealthy snacks. Additionally, missing breakfast may slow down the metabolism, making it harder for the body to efficiently burn calories.

Instead of skipping breakfast, consider opting for a balanced and nutritious morning meal to kickstart your metabolism, provide sustained energy, and set a positive tone for the rest of the day.

Importance of Nutrient-Dense Choices

The importance of nutrient-dense choices in breakfast cannot be overstated, especially when striving for weight loss. The concentration of vital vitamins, minerals, and other beneficial components in a food item relative to its calorie content is referred to as nutrient density. Choosing nutrient-dense foods for breakfast provides numerous benefits:

1. Sustained Energy:Nutrient-dense foods, such as whole grains, fruits, and lean proteins, release energy slowly, providing a sustained and steady source of fuel throughout the morning. This helps prevent energy crashes and the associated cravings for high-calorie snacks.

2. Supports Metabolism:
- Essential nutrients play a crucial role in supporting metabolic functions. Adequate intake of vitamins and minerals aids in the efficient utilization of calories, promoting a healthy metabolism.
3. Enhances Fullness and Satiety:

- Nutrient-dense foods are often rich in fiber and protein, both of which contribute to a feeling of fullness and satiety. This can help control appetite and reduce the likelihood of overeating later in the day.

4. Balanced Nutrition:-
- Nutrient-dense choices contribute to a well-balanced diet, ensuring that the body receives the necessary vitamins and minerals for optimal functioning. A healthy diet promotes general health and well-being.

5. Improved Nutrient Absorption:
- Nutrient-dense foods contain a variety of compounds that can enhance the absorption of essential nutrients. For example, pairing vitamin C-rich fruits with iron-containing foods can enhance iron absorption.

6. Promotes Long-Term Health:
- Consistently choosing nutrient-dense foods is associated with long-term health benefits. A diet rich in essential nutrients supports various bodily functions, reduces the risk of chronic diseases, and fosters overall well-being.
7. Optimizes Weight Loss Efforts:

-When aiming for weight loss, focusing on nutrient-dense choices allows individuals to achieve their calorie goals while still providing the necessary nutrients. This ensures that the body receives the nutrition it needs even with a reduced calorie intake.

8. Encourages Mindful Eating:
- Nutrient-dense foods often have more complex flavors and textures, encouraging a more mindful and enjoyable eating experience. This can lead to greater satisfaction with meals and reduced mindless snacking

In summary, prioritizing nutrient-dense choices for breakfast is a fundamental aspect of a healthy and effective weight loss strategy. It not only supports immediate goals but also contributes to long-term health and well-being. Making intentional and informed choices about the quality of the foods consumed at breakfast sets a positive tone for the entire day.

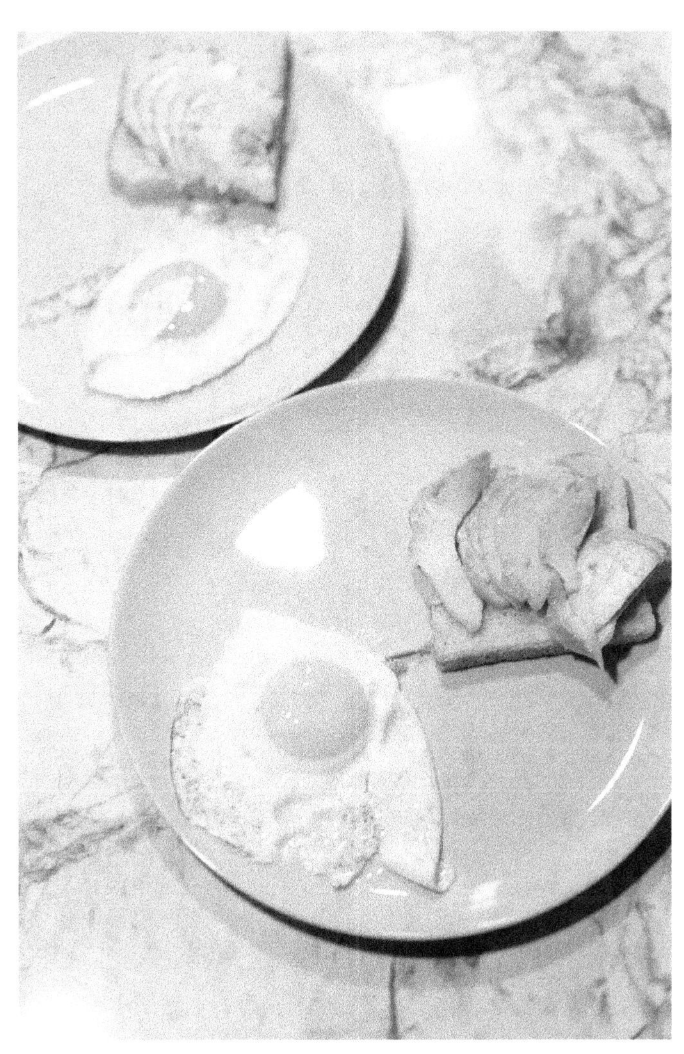

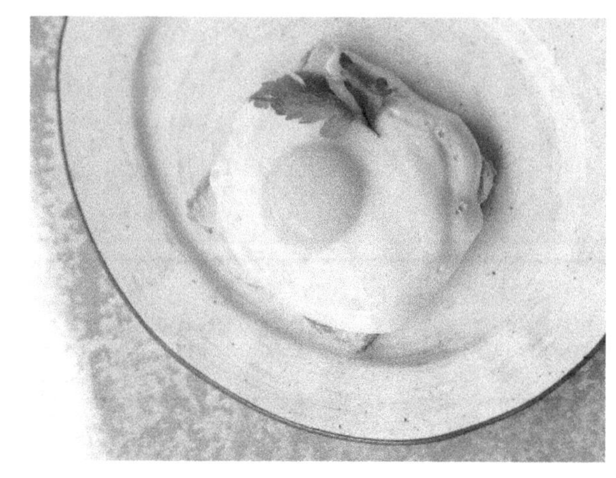

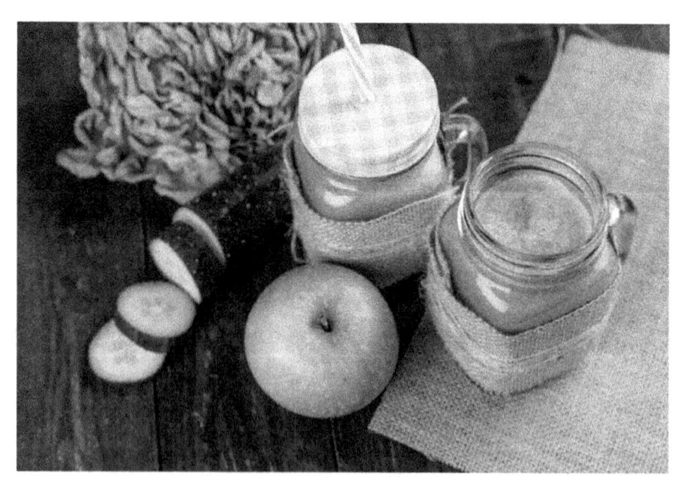

CHAPTER TWO

Important of breakfast for weight loss

Breakfast holds a pivotal role in weight loss for several reasons. Firstly, it jumpstarts your metabolism after a night of fasting, helping your body burn calories more efficiently throughout the day. By providing essential nutrients early on, breakfast sets the tone for a balanced diet, reducing the likelihood of overeating later.

A well-rounded breakfast stabilizes blood sugar levels, preventing energy crashes and cravings that often lead to unhealthy snacking. Choosing nutrient-dense foods in the morning can enhance satiety, making it easier to stick to portion control and make healthier food choices throughout the day.

Moreover, a wholesome breakfast can positively influence mood and cognitive function, fostering better decision-making when it comes to food. This combination of physiological and psychological benefits makes breakfast a valuable tool in achieving and maintaining weight loss goals.

In essence, a nutritious breakfast isn't just the first meal of the day; it's a strategic step toward a healthier lifestyle, providing the fuel and mindset needed to support weight loss efforts.

A healthy diet plays a crucial role in achieving and maintaining weight loss. Here are some key benefits:

- Calorie Control: A healthy diet helps control calorie intake, ensuring that you consume an appropriate amount for your weight loss goals. Nutrient-dense foods allow you to feel satisfied with fewer calories.

- Nutrient Density: Healthy foods are rich in essential nutrients, providing the body with vitamins, minerals, and antioxidants. This supports overall well-being and ensures that your body receives the necessary nutrients even when reducing calorie intake.

- Metabolism Boost: Certain foods can boost metabolism, aiding in the efficient burning of calories. For example, foods high in protein require more energy to digest, contributing to a higher metabolic rate.

- Blood Sugar Regulation: A balanced diet helps regulate blood sugar levels, preventing spikes and crashes. This stabilizes energy levels and reduces cravings for sugary, high-calorie snacks.

- Satiety and Portion Control: Nutrient-rich foods contribute to a feeling of fullness and satisfaction, reducing the likelihood of overeating. This supports portion control and helps in managing overall caloric intake.

- Muscle Preservation: A healthy diet, particularly one with sufficient protein, supports muscle preservation during weight loss. This is essential for maintaining a healthy metabolism and achieving a toned physique.

- Long-term Sustainability: Healthy eating habits are more sustainable in the long run, promoting a lifestyle change rather than a temporary diet. This sustainable approach is crucial for maintaining weight loss over time.

- Improved Digestion: Fiber-rich foods, such as fruits, vegetables, and whole grains, promote healthy digestion. This not only contributes to overall well-being but also aids in weight management by preventing constipation and bloating.

- Heart Health: A nutritious diet can improve cardiovascular health by reducing cholesterol levels and blood pressure. This is important for overall health and complements weight loss efforts.

- Emotional Well-being: Certain foods, such as those rich in omega-3 fatty acids, are associated with improved mood and mental well-being. Emotional stability can positively impact adherence to a weight loss plan.

In summary, a healthy diet is a multifaceted approach to weight loss, addressing not only calorie intake but also nutrient quality, metabolism, and overall well-being. Adopting a sustainable and balanced eating pattern is key to achieving and maintaining weight loss goals.

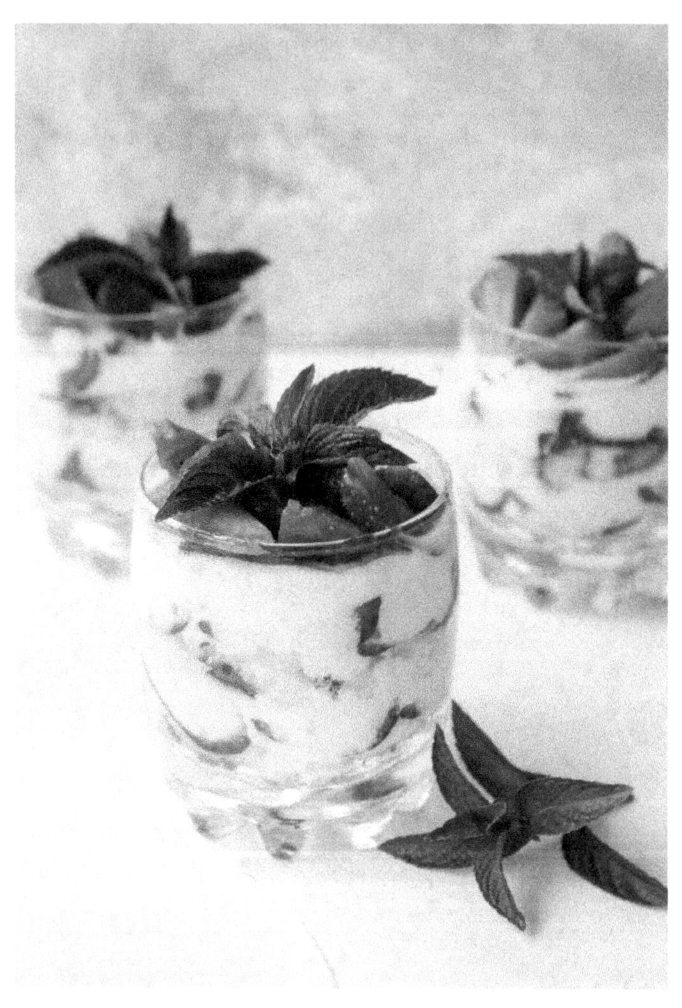

CHAPTER THREE

The principles of a healthy breakfast for weight loss

The principles of a healthy breakfast for weight loss revolve around making nutritious choices that provide essential nutrients while supporting calorie control. Here are key principles to consider:

1. Balance Macronutrients: Include a combination of carbohydrates, protein, and healthy fats in your breakfast. This balance helps maintain stable blood sugar levels, promotes satiety, and provides sustained energy throughout the morning.

2. Choose Whole Foods: Opt for minimally processed, whole foods such as fruits, vegetables, whole grains, lean proteins, and nuts. These foods are rich in nutrients and fiber, supporting overall health and aiding in weight loss.

3. Prioritize Protein: Protein-rich foods like eggs, Greek yogurt, lean meats, or plant-based sources like tofu can enhance feelings of fullness and help preserve muscle mass during weight loss.

4. Include Fiber: Foods high in fiber, such as whole grains, fruits, and vegetables, contribute to satiety and support digestive health. They also help regulate blood sugar levels, reducing the likelihood of energy crashes and cravings.

5. Limit Added Sugar: Minimize the intake of added sugars in breakfast items. Opt for natural sources of sweetness, such as fruits, and choose whole foods over sugary cereals or pastries.

6. Control Portions: Be mindful of portion sizes to avoid overeating. Even nutritious foods can contribute to excess calorie intake if consumed in large quantities.

7. Hydrate: Start your day with water or herbal tea to stay hydrated. Proper hydration benefits overall health and can aid with appetite management.

8. Include Nutrient-Dense Foods: Choose foods that provide a high amount of nutrients relative to their calorie content. This ensures that you get essential vitamins and minerals without excessive calories.

9. Limit Processed Foods: Minimize the consumption of processed and highly refined foods. These often lack nutritional value and may contribute to excess calorie intake.

10. Personalize Your Breakfast: Consider individual preferences, dietary restrictions, and cultural influences when planning your breakfast. Personalization increases the likelihood of adherence to a healthy eating plan.

11. Plan Ahead: Prepare breakfast items in advance to avoid unhealthy, impulsive choices on busy mornings. Planning allows you to make intentional, nutritious decisions.

By following these principles, a healthy breakfast becomes a cornerstone of a weight loss strategy, providing the necessary nutrients while aligning with overall health goals. Remember that a sustainable and enjoyable approach to breakfast is more likely to lead to long-term success in weight management.

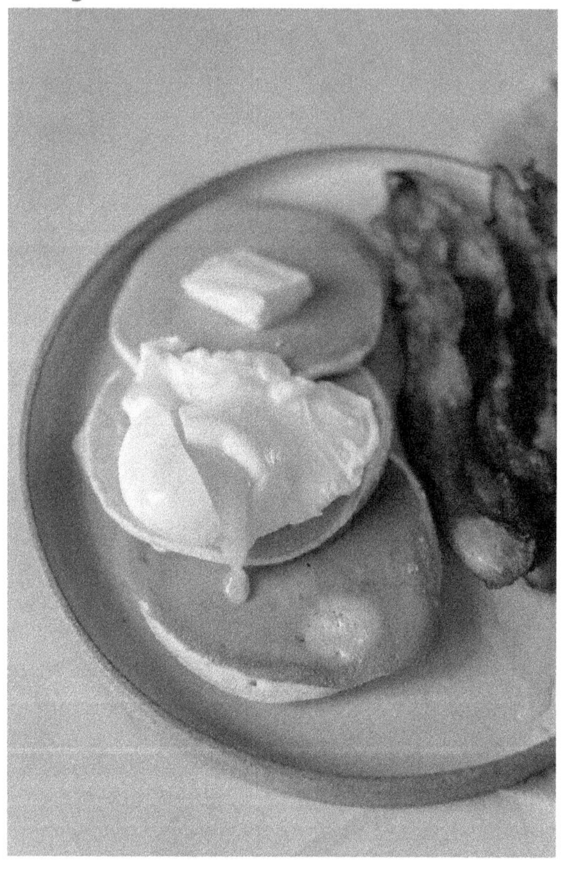

CHAPTER FOUR

Protein-packed breakfast ideas

1. Greek Yogurt Parfait:
   - Ingredients: Greek yogurt, mixed berries, granola, and honey drizzle.
   - Benefits: High protein from Greek yogurt, antioxidants from berries, and added crunch from granola.

2. Egg and Veggie Omelette:
   - Ingredients: Eggs, spinach, tomatoes, bell peppers, and a sprinkle of feta cheese.
   - Benefits: Protein-packed eggs combined with a variety of vegetables for added nutrients.

3. Protein Smoothie:
   - Ingredients: Protein powder, almond milk, banana, and a spoonful of nut butter.
   - Benefits: Quick and easy, customizable with different flavors, and provides a substantial protein boost.

4. Quinoa Breakfast Bowl:
- Ingredients: Cooked quinoa, Greek yogurt, sliced almonds, and fresh fruit (e.g berries or mango).
- Benefits: Quinoa is a complete protein, and the combination with Greek yogurt and nuts adds extra protein and texture.

5. Cottage Cheese and Fruit Plate:
- Ingredients: Cottage cheese, pineapple chunks, and a handful of sliced strawberries.
- Benefits: Cottage cheese is a rich source of protein, and pairing it with fresh fruit adds sweetness and vitamins.

6. Smoked Salmon Bagel:
- Ingredients: Whole grain bagel, smoked salmon, cream cheese, and capers.
- Benefits: Salmon is a lean protein source rich in omega-3 fatty acids, and the whole grain bagel adds fiber.

7. Chia Seed Pudding:

- Ingredients: Chia seeds, almond milk, vanilla extract, and topped with sliced almonds and berries.
- Benefits: Chia seeds are high in protein and omega-3 fatty acids, creating a satisfying and nutritious pudding.

8. Turkey and Avocado Wrap:
- Ingredients: Whole grain wrap, turkey slices, avocado, lettuce, and tomato.
- Benefits: Lean protein from turkey, healthy fats from avocado, and the wrap adds fiber.

9. Protein Pancakes:
- Ingredients: Protein pancake mix or homemade with protein powder, eggs, and oats.
- Benefits: A tasty and protein-packed alternative to traditional pancakes.

10. Soy Milk Smoothie Bowl:
- Ingredients: Soy milk, frozen mixed berries, banana, and a scoop of plant-based protein powder.

- Benefits: Plant-based protein from soy milk and protein powder, along with the goodness of berries.

These protein-packed breakfast ideas not only help meet your protein needs but also provide a delicious and satisfying start to your day.

How each protein packed breakfast are made

How each protein packed breakfast are made

Here are simple instructions for preparing each of the protein-packed breakfast ideas:

1. Greek Yogurt Parfait:
- In an empty glass or bowl, layer Greek yogurt, mixed berries, and granola.
- Drizzle honey on top for sweetness.

2. Egg and Veggie Omelette:
- Whisk the eggs and pour them into a hot nonstick pan.
- Add spinach, tomatoes, bell peppers, and feta cheese.

- Fold the omelette in half before serving.

3. Protein Smoothie:
   - Blend protein powder, almond milk, banana, and nut butter until smooth.
   - Adjust the consistency where necessary by adding more liquid.

4. Quinoa Breakfast Bowl:
   - Mix cooked quinoa with Greek yogurt.
   - Top with sliced almonds and fresh fruit like berries or mango.

5. Cottage Cheese and Fruit Plate:
   - Arrange cottage cheese on a plate.
   - Add pineapple chunks and sliced strawberries on top.

6. Smoked Salmon Bagel:
   - Toast a whole grain bagel.
   - Spread cream cheese on the bagel halves and top with smoked salmon and capers.

7. Chia Seed Pudding:
   - Mix chia seeds with almond milk and vanilla extract.

- Refrigerate overnight, then top with sliced almonds and berries before serving.

8. Turkey and Avocado Wrap:
- Lay out a whole grain wrap.
- Add turkey slices, avocado, lettuce, and tomato.
- Roll and cut the wrap in half.

9. Protein Pancakes:
- Mix protein pancake mix or a batter made from protein powder, eggs, and oats.
- Cook pancakes on a griddle until golden brown on both sides.

10. Soy Milk Smoothie Bowl:
- Blend soy milk, frozen mixed berries, banana, and plant-based protein powder until smooth.
- Pour into a bowl and add toppings like sliced banana and granola.

These recipes are designed to be simple and quick, making it easier to incorporate protein-packed breakfasts into your routine. Adjust the ingredients and quantities based on your preferences and dietary needs.

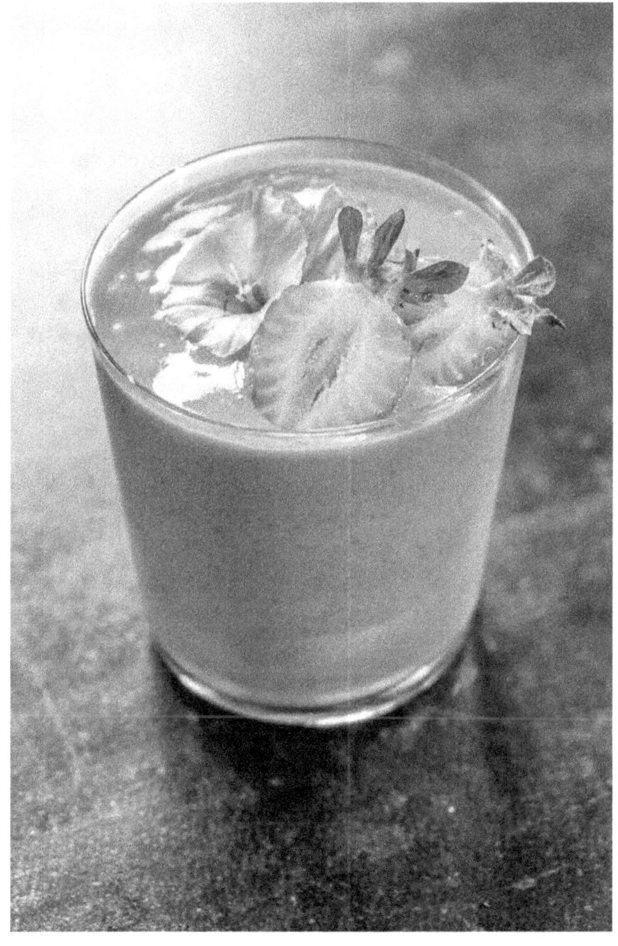

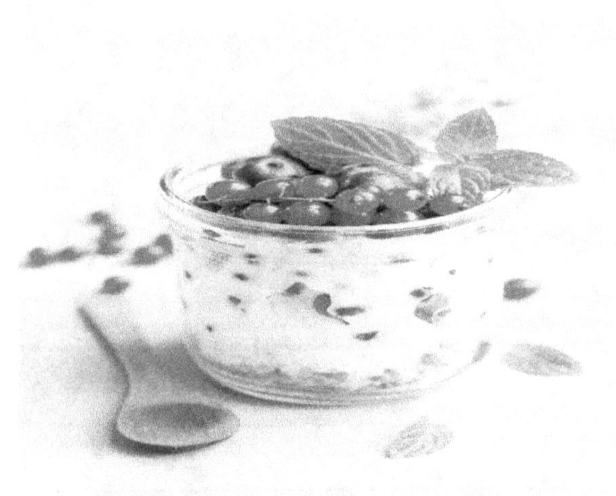

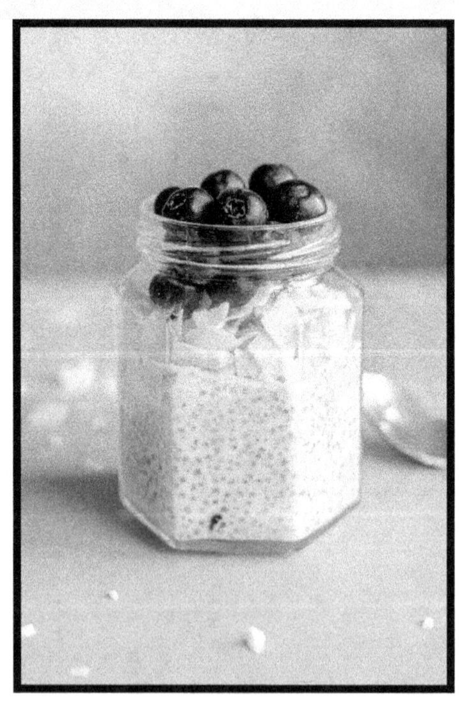

CHAPTER FIVE

WHOLE GRAIN BREAKFAST IDEAS

Here are some healthy and tasty whole grain breakfast ideas:

1. Oatmeal with Fresh Fruit:
   - Cook rolled oats in either water or milk.
   - Garnish with berries that are fresh, a diced banana, and nuts or seeds to serve.

2. Whole Wheat Toast with Avocado:
   - Toast whole wheat bread slices.
   - Incorporate with a little pepper and salt and top with fresh avocado.

3. Whole Grain Cereal with Yogurt:
   - Choose a fiber-rich whole grain cereal.
   - Serve with Greek yogurt and the berries of your choice.

4. Quinoa Breakfast Bowl:
   - Cook quinoa and combine it with the almond milk.

- Top with sliced almonds, diced mango, and honey drizzle.

5. Brown Rice Pudding:
   - Make brown rice by cooking it with milk, a little honey, and cinnamon.
   - Top with chopped nuts or raisins and serve warm.

6. Whole Grain Pancakes:
   - Use whole wheat flour or a combination of whole wheat and regular flour to make pancakes.
   - Add some fresh fruit or Greek yogurt on top.

7. Toast a whole grain in a bagel and top it with smoked salmon:
   - Cover each half with a layer of cream cheese, then garnish with red onion, capers, and smoked salmon.

8. Barley Breakfast Bowl:
   - Cook barley and mix with almond milk.
   - Add sliced peaches, a drizzle of maple syrup, and a sprinkle of chia seeds.

9. Whole Wheat English Muffin with Peanut Butter:
- Toast a whole wheat English muffin.
- Spread natural peanut butter on each half.

10. Muesli with Milk:
- Combine rolled oats, nuts, seeds, and dried fruit to make muesli.
- Soak in milk or yogurt overnight and enjoy in the morning.

11. Buckwheat Pancakes:
- Use buckwheat flour to make hearty pancakes.
- Serve with a dollop of yogurt and fresh berries.

12. Whole Grain Breakfast Burrito:
- Put scrambled eggs, black beans, salsa, and shredded cheese inside a whole grain tortilla.

In order to keep you energized throughout the morning, these whole grain breakfast ideas provide a good balance of fiber, vitamins, and minerals. Tailor them to your dietary restrictions and personal taste preferences.

The following are easy recipes for all the whole grain breakfast ideas:

1. Oatmeal with Fresh Fruit:
    - Follow the directions on the package to cook rolled oats with milk or water.
    - Add sliced banana, fresh berries, and a scattering of nuts or seeds on top.

2. Avocado on Whole Wheat Toast:
    - Toast some whole wheat bread slices.
    - Spread a mashed, ripe avocado over the toast.
    - To taste, add more salt and pepper.

3. Whole Grain Cereal with Yogurt:
    - Pick a high-fiber whole grain cereal.
    - After putting cereal in a bowl, top with Greek yogurt.
    - Place a few of your on top.

4. Quinoa Breakfast Bowl:
  * Cook quinoa according to package instructions.
  * Mix cooked quinoa with almond milk.
  * Top with sliced almonds, diced mango, and a drizzle of honey.

5. Brown Rice Pudding:
  * Cook brown rice with milk, cinnamon, and a touch of honey until creamy.
  * Serve warm, topped with raisins or chopped nuts.

6. Whole Grain Pancakes:
  * Mix whole wheat flour (or a mix of whole wheat and regular flour) with milk, eggs, and a pinch of baking powder.
  * Cook pancakes on a griddle until golden brown on both sides.
  * Top with fresh fruit or Greek yogurt.

7. Whole Grain Bagel with Smoked Salmon
  * Toast a whole grain bagel.
  * Spread cream cheese on each half.
  * Top with smoked salmon, capers, and red slices.

8. Barley Breakfast Bowl:
- Cook barley according to package instructions and mix with almond milk.
- Add sliced peaches, a drizzle of maple syrup, and a sprinkle of chia seeds.

9. Whole Wheat English Muffin with Peanut Butter:
- Toast a whole wheat English muffin.
- Spread natural peanut butter on each half.

10. Muesli with Milk:
- Combine rolled oats, nuts, seeds, and dried fruit to make muesli.
- Soak in milk or yogurt overnight, and enjoy in the morning.

11. Buckwheat flour, milk, eggs, and baking powder should be combined to make buckwheat pancakes.
- Pancakes should be griddle-cooked until golden brown.
- Present with some fresh berries and a dollop of yogurt.

12. Whole Grain Breakfast Burrito:
- Top scrambled eggs, black beans, salsa, and shredded cheese on a whole grain tortilla.
- After rolling, serve.

These recipes are designed to be straightforward, allowing you to enjoy a wholesome and satisfying whole grain breakfast. Adjust ingredients and quantities based on your preferences.

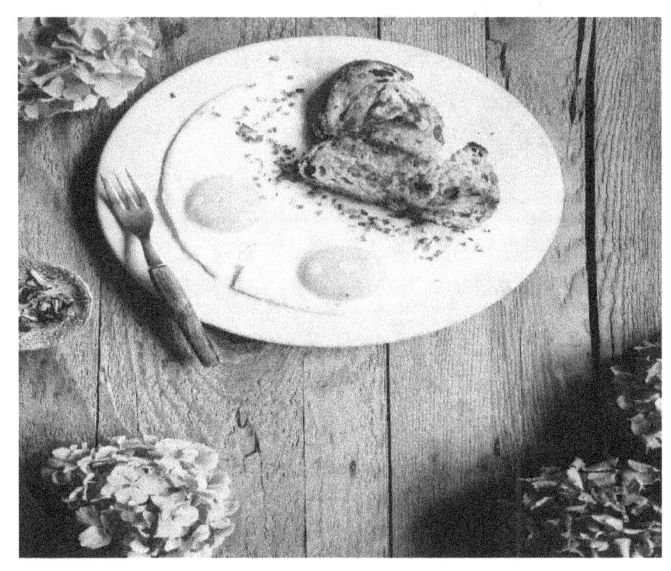

CHAPTER SIX

LOW CALORIES BREAKFAST IDEAS

Here are some low-calorie breakfast ideas that are both nutritious and delicious:

1. Egg White Omelette:
   - Whisk egg whites and cook with vegetables like spinach, tomatoes, and bell peppers. Season with herbs and spices.

2. Yogurt Parfait:
   - To add crunch, top nonfat Greek yogurt with a layer of fresh berries and granola.

3. Chia Seed Pudding:
   - Combine almond milk, chia seeds, and a small amount of vanilla extract. Put in the fridge for the night, then in the morning, top with sliced strawberries.

4. Vegetable Smoothie:

- Blend spinach, cucumber, celery, and a green apple for a refreshing and low-calorie green smoothie.

5. Cottage Cheese with Pineapple:
   - Combine low-fat cottage cheese with fresh pineapple chunks for a protein-rich and satisfying breakfast.

6. Light Whole Grain Toast:
   - Toast a slice of whole grain bread and top with a thin layer of almond butter or a slice of tomato.

7. Berries and Almond Milk Smoothie:
   - Blend mixed berries with unsweetened almond milk for a low-calorie, antioxidant-rich smoothie.

8. Veggie Scramble:
   - Cook a mixture of diced vegetables like zucchini, mushrooms, and cherry tomatoes with a touch of olive oil. Add scrambled eggs or egg whites.

9. Protein Pancakes:
   - Make pancakes using a mix of protein powder, egg whites, and a mashed banana. Top with a few blueberries.

10. Light Avocado Toast:
    - Top whole grain toast with a thin layer of mashed avocado. Add a pinch of red pepper flakes, salt, and pepper.
11. Low-Calorie Cereal Bowl:
    - Combine skim milk with a low-fat, high-fiber cereal. Add some berries or banana slices.
12. Steamed Asparagus with Poached Egg:
    - Steam asparagus spears and top with a poached egg. Season with salt, pepper, and a squeeze of lemon.

These breakfast ideas are not only low in calories but also provide essential nutrients to kickstart your day. Utilize serving sizes to your unique dietary requirements and preferences.

BENEFITS OF LOW-CALORIE BREAKFASTS:

Weight Management: Low-calorie breakfasts can contribute to overall calorie control, supporting weight management goals.

Nutrient Density: These breakfasts often pack a nutritional punch with vitamins, minerals, and other essential nutrients relative to their calorie content.

Improved Metabolism: Consuming a balanced, low-calorie breakfast can kickstart your metabolism, helping your body efficiently burn calories throughout the day.

Stable Blood Sugar: Low-calorie, nutrient-dense breakfasts can help regulate blood sugar levels, reducing energy crashes and sugar cravings.

Satiety: Despite being low in calories, these breakfasts are designed to be satisfying, helping you stay full until your next meal.

Don't forget to modify these suggestions according to your dietary requirements and preferences. Always consult with a healthcare professional or a nutritionist for personalized advice.

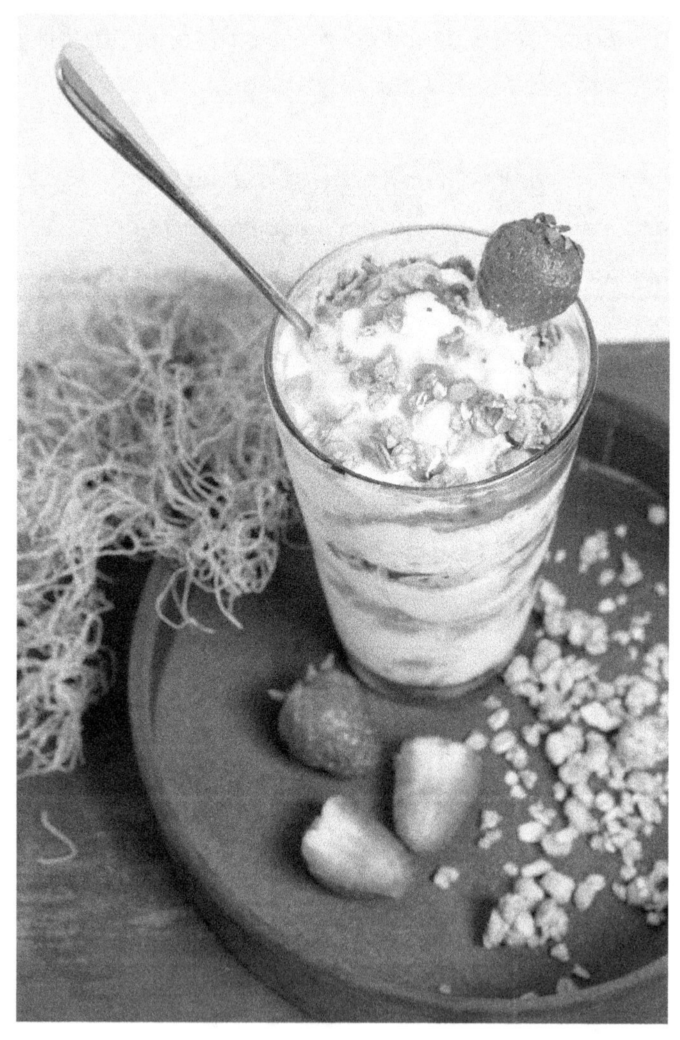

In conclusion, " Easy Breakfast Ideas for Weight Loss" serves as your compass on the path to a healthier and more vibrant life. With a plethora of mouthwatering recipes and insightful guidance, this book transforms the mundane task of breakfast into a delightful ritual that supports your weight loss journey. By embracing the principles of nutritious and satisfying morning meals, you are not just adopting a diet – you are cultivating a sustainable lifestyle.

So, turn the pages, savor the flavors, and let "Easy Breakfast Ideas for Weight Loss for beginners" be your trusted companion in the pursuit of well-being. Through the power of a wholesome breakfast, you're not just nourishing your body; you're igniting a positive change that ripples throughout your day and beyond. Start each morning with intention, flavor, and the knowledge that you hold the key to your own health. "Easy Breakfast Ideas for Weight Loss for beginners" is not just a book; it's an invitation to embrace a new dawn of wellness— one delicious bite at a time.

* 9 7 9 8 8 7 1 7 2 9 4 2 7 *